Practice Test 1

Practice Questions

1. Which of the following is NOT considered personal protective equipment?
    a. Gloves
    b. Gowns or other outer clothing
    c. Hand washing equipment
    d. Masks, face shields, goggles, and glasses

2. Which of the following terms expresses the ethical principle of doing good for the patient or others?
    a. Nonmaleficence
    b. Beneficence
    c. Veracity
    d. Confidentiality

3. When bathing a patient, the nursing aide should NOT:
    a. Wash the dirtiest area first
    b. Use standard precautions
    c. Use an assistive device
    d. Apply nonprescription ointments afterwards

4. At what point is cognitive dysfunction considered dementia?
    a. Anytime an individual experiences problems with memory, language, or problem solving
    b. When an individual has had memory, language, and problem-solving difficulties for over six months
    c. When a person has depression along with some memory loss
    d. When bodily functions as well as cognition are impaired

5. You observe a low respiration rate less than 12 breaths per minute in a patient. What could be the cause?
    a. The patient is in pain or under stress
    b. The patient is in respiratory distress
    c. The patient is taking narcotics
    d. The patient has an infection

6. Your patient refuses to see certain visitors, is withdrawn, and shows signs of bruising. What should you do?
    a. Mention this to the nurse
    b. Try to get the patient to see the aforementioned visitors
    c. Report suspected abuse according to facility policy
    d. Talk to the patient about his/her fears

7. Which of the following is NOT a reason to do range-of-motion exercises with a patient?
    a. To protect his/her muscles from atrophy, maintain joint motion, and increase circulation
    b. To lessen the likelihood of pressure ulcers
    c. To maintain mobility
    d. To normalize his/her vital signs

8. To whom should you report as a nursing assistant/nurse aide?
    a. A licensed physician
    b. The registered nurse or licensed practical nurse on your service
    c. The administrative desk person at the facility
    d. The professional assigning a particular task, which may be an RN, LPN, physical therapist, dietician, etc.

9. What should you do if you make a mistake in charting patient information?
    a. Start another chart
    b. Draw a single line in blue or black ink through the error, label it "error," and initial the mistake
    c. Use correction fluid over the error
    d. Have the supervising nurse write in a correction

10. What measures should you employ in order to communicate with a patient whose primary language is not English?
    a. Utilize a family member or other interpreter as an intermediary, and familiarize yourself with and honor his/her cultural perceptions of communication
    b. Let someone who speaks the patient's primary language communicate with him/her and report back to you
    c. Communicate primarily nonverbally through gestures, facial expressions, etc.
    d. Defer and have another aide who speaks his/her language assigned

11. What should you do if you find that a patient has fallen on the floor but does not appear to be hurt?
    a. Help the patient up and assist him/her back to bed
    b. Write a note to your supervisor
    c. Fill out an incident report that correctly records what happened and file it with the facility's risk manager
    d. Tell an administrator about the conditions that led to the fall

12. Which of the following should NOT be done when caring for a patient with an indwelling catheter?
    a. The patient should be positioned on his/her side
    b. The urethra should be cleansed using a downward circular motion
    c. The bag should be hung below the level of the bladder, but not touching the floor
    d. The tubing should be fixed firmly to the person's inner thigh

13. What is the best way to provide for your patient's spiritual needs?
    a. Refer him/her to some type of religious counselor
    b. Alert him/her to religious services in the facility
    c. Establish rapport with the patient and find out about his/her spiritual needs and views on spirituality
    d. Pray with the patient

- 4 -

14. What should be suspected if a patient being treated for pain experiences a sudden drop in blood pressure, a change in respiration, and the appearance of a rash?
    a. Anxiety or stress
    b. Fluid loss
    c. An adverse drug effect from the analgesic
    d. Hypertension

15. Under what circumstances should a nursing aide have access to a patient's files?
    a. A nursing aide can access files on any patient that he/she has cared for
    b. A nursing aide can access files on patients currently under his/her care
    c. A nursing aide can access files in order to show information to family members
    d. A nursing aide can access files in order to correct computer information

16. Which of the following is a good method of communicating with a patient?
    a. Keep the conversation light and questions short
    b. Maintain eye contact, speak slowly using laymen's terms, and try to ask open-ended questions
    c. Be authoritative, letting the patient know your expertise
    d. Always be assuring

17. What should you do if a patient who is ambulating with your help and a gait belt begins to fall?
    a. Try to prevent the fall by any means
    b. Change your position to block the fall
    c. Keep your feet wide apart, bend your knees, lower the patient to the floor, and then let him/her rest on your leg
    d. Let the patient fall and then, using good body mechanics, pick him/her back up

18. Which of the following is incorrect regarding placing a vest (jacket) restraint on a patient?
    a. A doctor's order and family consent must be obtained beforehand
    b. The straps should be tied to a chair or the bed frame with a quick-release knot
    c. The distance between the chest and the vest should be about the width of two fingers
    d. The opening and straps should be across the front

19. What should you do if a patient makes a blatant sexual comment to you?
    a. Counter with sexual remarks of your own
    b. Firmly but politely inform him/her that these types of comments are unacceptable and will not be tolerated
    c. Immediately inform your supervisor
    d. Ignore the behavior

20. How does the right to informed consent impact nursing home residents?
    a. Since they may be incapacitated, it does not apply
    b. Informed consent must be obtained from the residents or their health care power of attorney prior to every test, treatment, or procedure
    c. It prevents them from changing or stopping treatments once a decision has been made
    d. Its applicability is broader than in other circumstances

21. You badger a patient into allowing you to give him/her a bath with the door open. Of what legally liable acts could you possibly be accused?
    a. Assault and battery
    b. Abuse
    c. Invasion of privacy
    d. Assault, battery, invasion of privacy, and abuse

22. What is the most likely isolation scenario for a patient who has MRSA?
    a. Placement of the patient in a clearly marked private room, and wearing by the nurse aide (and others) of an isolation gown and gloves at all times while in the room
    b. Same precautions as choice A (above) plus wearing a mask
    c. Placement of the patient in a negative pressure room and use by the nurse aide of a mask or respirator and gloves while in the room
    d. Isolation of the patient in a separate ward with other MRSA patients

23. Which of the following are signs that your patient is dehydrated?
    a. He/she has peripheral edema, bulging veins, and lung crackles
    b. He/she has cloudy urine and flank pain
    c. He/she has a weak, fast pulse, low blood pressure, dark urine, and sunken eyes
    d. He/she is constipated

24. What are the primary responsibilities of a nursing assistant in a code situation?
    a. To assist other personnel when asked
    b. To get any needed equipment and if certified, to provide relief CPR if necessary
    c. The nursing assistant plays no role in a code situation.
    d. To stand outside the room and allow only appropriate personnel inside

25. For what type of patients is the use of the logrolling technique appropriate?
    a. Patients from whom you need to obtain a urine specimen
    b. Patients capable of helping you to move them
    c. Patients in respiratory distress
    d. Patients who have sustained a neck or spinal cord injury

26. An electrical fire starts in your patient's room. What should you do?
    a. Immediately try to extinguish it with a type A fire extinguisher
    b. Remove the patient, activate the fire alarm, close doors, and use a type A fire extinguisher on the fire
    c. Immediately try to extinguish it with a type C or ABC fire extinguisher
    d. Remove the patient, activate the fire alarm, close doors, and use a type C or ABC fire extinguisher on the fire

27. Your patient has an area of skin that is somewhat worn away and red. What condition does he/she have?
    a. A skin allergy
    b. A stage II pressure sore
    c. A stage III pressure sore
    d. A stage IV pressure sore

28. What should you do if your patient insists upon seeing his/her chart?
    a. Tell the patient politely that you cannot show it to him/her
    b. Show the patient the chart
    c. Inform the charge nurse before showing the patient the chart
    d. Inform the charge nurse and contact medical records to make a copy of the chart to show the patient

29. Your patient has aphasia. Which of the following is NOT a possible cause?
    a. A cerebrovascular accident
    b. A brain tumor
    c. Diabetes
    d. Parkinson's disease

30. You take your patient's temperature and find it to be 97.3ºF. Which of the following could definitely NOT have caused this?
    a. The patient is starting to get an infection
    b. The patient has been resting
    c. The patient drank something within 15 minutes of an oral temperature reading
    d. The patient has recently come out of the operating room

31. What should you NEVER do if a patient insists on using the call light or bell whether or not he/she really needs to?
    a. Ignore the call light or bell if you are aware of this behavior
    b. Tape gauze over the call button
    c. Stop in as often as possible to talk to that patient
    d. Make sure the items the patient will need are readily available

32. Directives for what types of measures are generally covered on a DNR order?
    a. Organ/tissue donation after death
    b. Use of long-term mechanical ventilation, continuous dialysis, and/or a feeding tube
    c. Use of new intubation, CPR, and/or defibrillation if near death or unconscious
    d. Designation of another person to make medical decisions if the patient is unable to do so

33. How should a thermometer used for taking a resident's temperature be treated in terms of potential for infection?
    a. It should be sterilized between uses
    b. It should be treated with a high-level disinfectant between uses
    c. It should be cleaned with soap and rinsed between uses
    d. It should be wiped off between uses

34. Which of the following is NOT a possible treatment for a contracture?
    a. Use of a splint
    b. Range-of-motion exercises
    c. Use of a dressing
    d. Use of heat therapy

35. How does oral care for an unconscious patient differ from that for a conscious one?
    a. The unconscious patient should be placed in the Fowler's position
    b. A towel should be draped over the patient's chest
    c. A tongue depressor should be used to keep the patient's mouth open and suctioning should be done afterwards
    d. The aide should wear gloves during the procedure

36. Which of the following is ALWAYS outside the scope of practice of a nursing assistant?
    a. Insertion or removal of an indwelling catheter
    b. Administration of medications to the patient
    c. Helping the patient with self-administration of drugs
    d. Following the supervising nurse's orders

37. Which of the following should NOT be done for a patient who has Sundowner's syndrome?
    a. Promote daytime exercise
    b. Allow sleeping during the day
    c. Darken the room when it is time to sleep
    d. Give a therapeutic massage at night

38. If you have given a patient 4 ounces of juice, how should you report that on his/her chart?
    a. As 4 ounces of juice
    b. As a half cup of juice
    c. As 60 mL or cc of juice
    d. As 120 mL or cc of juice

39. What is h.s. care?
    a. Care provided at bedtime
    b. Washing of the patient's hair
    c. Care provided in the morning
    d. Bathing of the patient

40. What is the correct way to transfer a patient from the bed to a wheelchair?
    a. While you hold under the axilla, have the patient pivot into the chair from dangling on the side of the bed
    b. While you hold under the axilla, help the patient push down on the mattress from the side of the bed and stand up; then pivot and lower the patient into the wheelchair
    c. With another helper, lift the patient into the wheelchair
    d. Use the logrolling technique

41. What is the first stage of grief a person experiences after being informed that he/she is dying?
    a. Anger
    b. Denial
    c. Depression
    d. Acceptance

42. Which of the following changes is probably NOT a sign of impending death?
    a. Heart rate slows and becomes irregular
    b. Breathing sounds rattling or raspy
    c. Eyes flicker
    d. Blood pressure and core temperature decrease

- 8 -

43. How does taking an apical pulse differ from taking a peripheral pulse?
    a. An apical pulse is taken using the index and middle fingers over the hollow of the wrist
    b. An apical pulse reading utilizes auscultation with a stethoscope over the left chest
    c. Pressure is applied when taking an apical pulse
    d. An apical pulse is counted for a longer period of time

44. If you as a nursing assistant fail to perform or incorrectly perform procedures that you were taught, for what could you potentially be sued?
    a. Defamation
    b. Malpractice
    c. Neglect
    d. Negligence

45. Which of the following types of patients can include pork in their diet?
    a. Muslim
    b. Jewish
    c. Catholic
    d. Hindu

46. Which of the following is NOT a principle of good body mechanics to prevent injuries during lifting?
    a. Maintain good posture while lifting
    b. Stand with a wide base of support
    c. Bend over to pick up the person or object
    d. Maintain body alignment and keep items close to you

47. What type of information can a nursing assistant communicate to family members?
    a. Lab results
    b. The patient's prognosis
    c. Information about procedures within his/her own scope of practice
    d. Information about the overall care of the patient

48. Which of the following scenarios do NOT require you to do proper hand washing?
    a. You have just entered the patient's room but have not touched anyone or any surface
    b. You are getting ready to feed the patient
    c. You have just used the restroom
    d. You have come into contact with the patient's bodily fluids but were wearing gloves

49. Which of the following are typical requirements to become a certified nursing assistant?
    a. On-the-job training
    b. On-the-job training, recommendation by a supervisor, and passing an administered exam
    c. At least 75 hours of classroom and basic skills training, and passing a state certification exam including a written examination and a demonstration of skills
    d. At least 120 hours of classroom and basic skills training, and passing a state certification exam including a written examination and a demonstration of skills

50. When might an NPO diet be ordered for a patient?
   a. If the patient is diabetic
   b. When the patient is about to undergo some type of testing or surgical procedure, or if the patient is in a situation where he/she cannot swallow
   c. If the patient has hypertension
   d. If the patient has difficulty chewing

51. What is the correct sequence for removal of soiled linen from an isolation room?
   a. Put soiled linen in a plastic linen bag, tie the bag shut upon completion of bathing the patient, slip that bag into another one being held by another aide outside the door, other aide ties and leaves the double bag outside the door, remove personal protective equipment (PPE) and wash hands, take double bag to soiled utility area
   b. Put soiled linen in a plastic linen bag, tie the bag shut upon completion of bathing the patient, put bag outside door, remove PPE and wash hands, take bag to soiled utility area
   c. Put soiled linen in a plastic linen bag, tie bag shut and insert into another bag, leave double bag in room until several have been collected, take bags to soiled utility area
   d. Put linen in soiled utility bin in the room until full, double bag while using PPE, remove PPE and wash hands, take bag to soiled utility area

52. All EXCEPT which of the following might be utilized if a patient experiences redness, swelling, and pain in his/her leg?
   a. A sequential compression device
   b. Use of anticoagulants or surgery
   c. Massaging of the affected leg
   d. Anti-embolism stockings

53. What should you do if an alert, mentally capable patient expresses a wish to leave the health-care facility?
   a. Have the patient sign an Against Medical Advice form, and let him/her leave
   b. Notify the charge nurse who will talk to the patient and notify the doctor if the patient leaves
   c. Try to talk the patient out of doing so
   d. Notify the family to deal with the matter

54. What may dark, tarry stools indicate?
   a. Diarrhea
   b. Constipation
   c. Intestinal bleeding
   d. Dehydration

55. The capacity to understand what a patient is feeling and respond appropriately is known as what?
   a. Active listening
   b. Empathy
   c. Caring
   d. Respect

56. When you are making an occupied bed, what should be observed in terms of the orientation of the patient and the use of the side rails?
    a. The patient should be lying supine with the side rail down on the side of the bed you are making but up on the other side
    b. The patient should be lying on his/her side facing you with the side rail down on the side you are making but up on the other side
    c. The patient should be lying on his/her side facing away from you with the side rail down on the side you are making but up on the other side
    d. The patient should be lying supine and neither side rail should be lowered throughout

57. Which of the following procedures is NOT generally done as part of postmortem care?
    a. Closing of the patient's eyes and removal of lines and tubes
    b. All hygienic, grooming, and other procedures normally provided to a living patient
    c. Placing the patient in a supine position
    d. Placing the body in a plastic bag

58. How should you proceed if the Heimlich maneuver is needed on a choking patient?
    a. Stand behind the person, drape your arms around him/her, make a fist with your thumb toward the person just above the navel, grab that fist with the other hand, quickly and forcefully thrust in and up on the abdomen, repeating until the object dislodges
    b. Same as choice A (above) but if person becomes unconscious, check for respirations and pulse and do rescue breathing and/or CPR if necessary
    c. Same as choice A (above) but do the thrusts gently to avoid injuring the person
    d. Call emergency services immediately

59. What is the Patient's Bill of Rights?
    a. A federal law listing rights of hospitalized patients
    b. A federal act guaranteeing the privacy of patient health information
    c. A document given to an admitted patient or resident listing his/her responsibilities while staying in the facility
    d. A document given to an admitted patient or resident listing his/her rights while staying in the facility

60. Which of the following is an example of an unintentional tort?
    a. The nursing assistant checks out early without telling her supervisor and the patient falls out of bed and breaks a bone
    b. The nursing assistant inadvertently forgets to put up the side rails on a patient's bed and the patient falls out and breaks a bone
    c. The nursing assistant stabs a member of the patient's family
    d. The nursing assistant beats a patient unconscious

61. In what direction(s) should you wash and dry the perineal area of a female patient?
    a. You should wash from the front to the back going from the urinary meatus to vulva to perineum, rinse using a clean cloth, and then dry in the same front to back direction
    b. You should wash the same areas listed in choice A (above) from back to front, rinse using a clean cloth, and then dry from back to front
    c. You should wash and then rinse and dry the urinary meatus, then wash and dry the vulva, and then wash and dry the perineum
    d. You should wash and then rinse and dry the perineum, wash and then rinse and dry the vulva, and then wash and rinse and dry the urinary meatus

- 11 -

62. Which of the following scenarios is NOT a justifiable reason for you to refuse an assignment?
    a. You do not get along with the patient
    b. You feel that carrying out the requested task could endanger the patient or yourself
    c. The task is outside a nursing assistant's scope of practice
    d. You feel that you do not know how to perform the task

63. What are signs that your diabetic patient might have low blood sugar?
    a. The skin is hot and flushed, respirations are deep, pulse is slow, breath is fruity, and/or speech is garbled
    b. The patient is confused
    c. The skin is cold and sweaty, respirations are shallow, and pulse is rapid and barely perceptible
    d. The patient is very thirsty

64. How should you refer to a patient who has severe vision and hearing problems?
    a. Disabled
    b. Blind and deaf
    c. Vision-impaired and hearing-impaired
    d. Sightless and hard-of-hearing

65. When recording intake and output, what should be recorded as output?
    a. Urine and stool total output in milliliters (mL) or cubic centimeters (cc)
    b. All fluids secreted by the patient in mL or cc
    c. Urine output in mL or cc
    d. Urine output in ounces

66. A patient is wearing several pieces of valuable jewelry upon admission. Which of the following is NOT a proper way to deal with this situation?
    a. Ask the patient to give the jewelry to a family member to hold onto and take home
    b. Catalogue the jewelry and put it in a marked box in the hospital safe
    c. Give the patient a case to keep the jewelry in alongside his/her bed
    d. Bring in a witness if you handle the jewelry

67. When measuring blood pressure, where should the individual's arm be placed?
    a. Below the level of the heart
    b. At the level of the heart if seated and at his/her side if lying down
    c. Above the level of the heart
    d. Initially at the level of the heart and then lowered upon starting the cuff deflating sequence

68. What is continuity of care?
    a. Transfer of patient care from one facility to another
    b. Transfer of patient care to a provider on another shift
    c. A recognized standard of patient care
    d. A patient's right to and the caregiver's performance of continual and consistent high-quality health care

69. Your patient has poor lower body strength and fairly weak upper body strength as well. What is the best technique to use for ambulation on crutches?
    a. The three-point technique
    b. The four-point technique
    c. The swing-to method
    d. The swing-through method

70. What is the proper water temperature for a tub bath?
    a. 90°F
    b. 105°F
    c. 115°F
    d. 120°F

Answers and Explanations

1. C: Hand washing equipment is not personal protective equipment, but hand washing is a precaution for infection control and should be performed before donning and after removing gloves (A) and at many other times. Personal protective equipment (PPE), which should be worn whenever you may be in contact with blood and other bodily fluids, includes gloves (A); gowns or other removable outer clothing (B); and face protection (D) against splashes or airborne pathogens, including a mask and a face shield, goggles, or protective glasses.

2. B: These are all ethical principles, which are standards of correct moral conduct. Beneficence (B) is the correct term for doing good for others. Nonmaleficence (A) refers to the ethical principle of providing care that does not cause harm. Veracity (C) means speaking truthfully at all times. Confidentiality (D) is the code of maintaining the privacy of the patient's information.

3. A: When the aide is bathing the patient, he/she should wash starting with the cleanest area and progressing to the dirtiest. Bathing as well as grooming activities should employ standard precautions (B). Assistive devices (C) are not always used, but should be utilized for patients at high risk for falls. While prescription ointments must be applied by a licensed nurse, nonprescription emollients (D) can be applied sparingly afterwards by the aide.

4. B: When an individual experiences cognitive dysfunction such as loss of memory, language, and problem-solving ability for over six months, that is considered dementia. These losses for less than six months (A) are classified as delirium. Depression along with memory loss (C) does occur often with dementia but the combination alone is not definitive. Impairment of bodily functions in addition to cognitive dysfunction (D) is often an end stage for the most common form of dementia, Alzheimer's disease.

5. C: Use of narcotics can depress the respiratory drive and rate. A low rate (less than 12 breaths per minute) also can occur when at rest or lying on one's back. The other choices (as well as a heart attack and fluid overload) all generally result in an elevated respiratory rate.

6. C: These are signs of possible physical, sexual, and/or mental abuse, and therefore the aide has a moral, ethical, and legal obligation to inform authorities of his/her suspicions. It is not enough to merely inform the nurse (A), the issue is too sensitive to talk about with the patient (D), and the patient should not be encouraged to meet with the visitors who may be abusing him/her (B).

7. D: ROM exercises might, but do not directly, improve vital signs. Range-of-motion (ROM) or passive range-of-motion exercises (PROM) are actively or passively assisted exercises for maintaining joint mobility (C). They encourage all positive aspects associated with mobility, including prevention of muscle atrophy, increased joint motion, and better circulation (A); they decrease the likelihood of development of pressure ulcers (B); and they help reduce the propensity to develop respiratory infections, gastrointestinal problems, and osteoporosis.

8. B: A nursing assistant or nurse aide (CNA) is assigned duties by either a registered nurse (RN) or licensed practical nurse (LPN) under the RN, and the aide should generally report to the nurse. There may be situations when a licensed physician (A) is in charge, but usually an RN is employed to carry out the medical plan. It is inappropriate to report to administrators (C) or other professionals (D).

9. B: The only way for any professional to correct an error made on a chart is to draw a single line in blue or black ink, label it "error," and initial the mistake. Correction fluid (C) or erasing should not be used, another chart should not be started (A), and another professional such as the supervising nurse (D) should not intervene. Charting should include things like vital signs, assessments, and procedural commentary.

10. A: The nurse aide should be present to maintain contact with the patient through an interpreter and take into account the patient's cultural beliefs. For example, various cultures have different views on personal space or the appropriate physical distance to maintain. The aide should not leave while an interpreter talks to a patient (B), change patients (D), or use only nonverbal communication (C) which might be misinterpreted.

11. C: Whenever a fall occurs, the aide or other professional should fill out an incident report and convey it to the facility's risk manager, regardless of whether or not the person appears to be hurt. Merely writing a note to your supervisor (B) or telling an administrator (D) is not enough. You and another professional may end up helping the patient up and assisting him/her back to bed (A), but the report must be filed.

12. A: The patient should be in a supine position with the head of the bed lowered, not on his/her side. All of the other choices given should be part of the procedure. The aide should also wash his/her hands and use gloves, place a waterproof pad under the hips, and dry the perineal area when finished.

13. C: The nursing assistant should establish rapport with the patient and listen to his/her views about spirituality and spiritual needs. Spirituality is any means of finding inner meaning from life in order to feel completeness or self-actualization. It can be associated with established religion but can also come from other sources such as nature. If you find that the patient does have a particular religious affiliation that nurtures him/her, any of the other choices might be utilized.

14. C: The most likely cause is an adverse drug effect (ADE) due to administration of an analgesic drug for the pain, which should be immediately reported to the supervising nurse to address the emergency. A rash generally would not be associated with any of the other conditions. Dehydration from fluid loss (B) can adversely affect various bodily systems but since fluid intake and output should be monitored it is less likely. Conversely, hypertension (D), or high blood pressure, is often due to fluid overload. Anxiety (A) alone would not cause this combination of symptoms.

15. B: The patient has a right to confidentiality, which means that nursing aides or other professionals should only have access to files on patients currently under their care, not those they have previously cared for (A). Under the right to privacy, family members generally cannot access information unless they provide the patient's privacy code number; if they do not have this, the nursing assistant can only confirm the patient's presence (C). Legally, the nursing assistant should not be making computer changes (D).

16. B: This response lists some of the features of good communication, namely maintaining eye contact, using terms the individual can understand, and asking questions that are open-ended to encourage the person to give more information. A is incorrect because it negates the seriousness of the situation and encourages yes or no responses which lead nowhere. C is wrong because your role is to be supportive, not authoritative, and D is also wrong because you should not give the person false hope.

17. C: A patient using a gait belt to ambulate with your help generally needs minimum assistance, and this sequence is suggested if he/she begins to fall. You should not move the patient. Call for help, notify your supervisor, and file an incident report. The fall should not be prevented (A), blocked (B), or allowed to occur haphazardly (D).

18. D: The vest restraint opening and the straps crossing should both be behind the back, not in the front. Doctor and family permission must be obtained prior to using this type of restraint (A), the straps should be secured to a chair or the bed frame (B), and to permit breathing a distance of about the width of two fingers should be allowed (C).

19. B: You need to first let him/her know firmly and politely that these comments are unacceptable and cannot continue. If the behavior persists, then your supervisor should be notified (C). Joking or sexual responses are inappropriate (A), and the behavior should not be ignored and allowed to continue (D).

20. B: Just as with other types of patients, the right of informed consent applies and means that prior to performance of any test, treatment, or procedure, the patient or his/her representative must be informed of the risks and benefits so that he/she may consent or decline. That negates responses A and D. However, under the right of freedom of choice, the patient can later change or stop treatments (C).

21. D: You could possibly be accused of all of these acts: assault (the threat of touching without permission); battery (actual personal violence without permission); invasion of privacy (exposing the client's body during care or failure to maintain confidentiality); and abuse (threatened or actual physical or mental harm to the patient).

22. A: MRSA, methicillin-resistant *Staphylococcus aureus*, is primarily a bloodborne pathogen spread via direct contact, and therefore contact precautions as indicated in A should be used. Scenario B describes droplet precautions for microorganisms spread via mucous or respiratory secretions, while C expresses airborne precautions for organisms that can survive a long time in the environment. The patient probably would not be put in a separate ward (D) where he/she would be in contact with others.

23. C: These are all signs of dehydration, which indicate that fluids should be encouraged. Constipation (D) may be a sign of dehydration but could also be due to use of medications that reduce GI motility. Scenario A suggests fluid overload, and B suggests the presence of a urinary tract infection.

24. B: The nursing assistant's main role in a code situation is to get the equipment and, if certified, he/she might help provide CPR. He/she is not qualified to provide any other type of assistance (A). If the room is crowded, the assistant may move out of the way and near the door in order to hear instructions (D).

25. D: The logrolling technique, in which at least two caregivers turn the patient together toward them to a side-lying or Sims' position using a pull sheet, should be used with patients who have sustained a neck or spinal injury because it keeps those areas in a stable position, preventing further injury. These patients are not capable of assisting in the move (B), and there is no need to use the technique to obtain a urine specimen (A) or when a patient is in respiratory distress (C).

26. D: When any fire occurs, the RACE system illustrated in answers B and D should be utilized. In this case, a silver type A fire extinguisher (A or B) should not be used because it shoots water and is only appropriate for ordinary combustibles such as paper. Type C is red, discharges dry chemicals, and is appropriate for an electrical fire. Multipurpose type ABC is also red and can be used for fires involving combustibles, liquid chemicals, or electrical sources.

27. B: The patient has a stage II pressure sore. Both stage I and II pressure sores show areas of redness, but with stage II there is also wearing away of the outer layer of skin. Stage III sores are black and indicate wearing of the full thickness of skin, and with stage IV there is an exposed area of visible bone. Skin allergies generally are not characterized by skin loss.

28. D: The charge nurse should first be notified, but instead of showing the patient the actual chart (C or B), a copy should be obtained from medical records so that the actual chart cannot be altered. Patients are legally allowed to see the information in their chart, so A is wrong.

29. C: Diabetes is unrelated to the presence of aphasia, which is difficulty speaking due to brain lesions caused by factors such as a cerebrovascular accident (stroke, A), a brain tumor (B), progressive diseases such as Parkinson's or Alzheimer's (D), or brain injury.

30. B: At rest, a person who is otherwise healthy should have a normal core temperature of between 97.8°F and 99.1°F. While elevated temperature generally indicates infection, initially a person could have a low core temperature (A). If the method of taking temperature is oral, the reading should not be taken within 15 minutes of drinking as that can lower the value (C). Operating rooms can be cold and thus lower core temperature temporarily (D).

31. A: You should never ignore a call light or bell, regardless of assumed patient behavior. Item B is actually a means by which the patient can find the correct button if he/she needs to call the aide or nurse. C and D are ways of hopefully cutting down on use of the call light or bell.

32. C: Directions for use of the heroic measures listed in C are part of a Do Not Resuscitate (DNR) order. Items A and B are addressed in an advanced directive regarding end-of-life care, and item D refers to designation of a medical durable power of attorney.

33. B: Even if it is covered with a plastic probe cover, a thermometer would be considered an intermediate-risk item that comes in contact with mucous membranes but does not penetrate the skin, and as such should be cleaned with a high-level disinfectant. Even if it does pierce the skin, a thermometer really cannot undergo sterilization procedures (A) appropriate for high-risk items like surgical instruments. C is appropriate for low-risk items, and D is insufficient for anything touching skin.

34. C: A contracture is an area of muscle tightening, which is a problem when it affects joint motion. Therefore, a splint for stretching the joint (A), range-of-motion exercises (B), and heat (D) are all helpful, but there is no need for a dressing.

35. C: The unique parts of oral care for an unconscious patient are keeping the mouth open with a tongue depressor and use of suctioning afterwards. All patients should receive oral care in the Fowler's position (head of bed elevation of 30 to 90 degrees, A) with a towel over the chest (B) and use of gloves by the aide (D).

36. A: Insertion or removal of a device such as an indwelling catheter (or performance of any sterile procedure) is outside the nursing assistant's scope of practice and could result in liability for the action. Choices B and C having to do with administration of drugs are usually outside the scope of practice but may be allowed in some states or instances *if* the assistant has received special training. Following a supervising nurse's orders (D) is a normal part of the nursing assistant's daily duties.

37. B: The patient with Sundowner's syndrome gets confused or agitated in late afternoon or early evening. The syndrome may or may not be associated with dementia. The patient should not be allowed to sleep during the day since he/she will have more difficulty sleeping at night. All of the other actions are generally helpful.

38. D: Fluid measurements should be reported as mL (milliliters) or cc (cubic centimeters). Since the conversion factor is 30 mL per ounce, the correct answer is 120 mL or cc.

39. A: The term h.s. care stands for hour of sleep care provided at night. It includes a condensed version of skin care with washing of the face and hands, oral care, and possibly a back rub. Care provided in the morning (C) is termed a.m. care and is more extensive, including a full bath, shaving, dressing, and hair, oral, and nail care. The other choices are part of providing for activities of daily living but are incorrect.

40. B: The patient should be assisted to stand up first, not to directly pivot to sit in the wheelchair (A). Wheels on the bed and wheelchair should be locked. The other responses are incorrect.

41. B: There are five stages in the grieving process, the first being denial. Subsequent stages in order are anger (A), bargaining, depression (C), and acceptance (D).

42. C: Flickering or other unique eye movements are not associated with impending death, but all the other signs listed are, as well as depression of respiratory rhythm and rate, cyanotic lips, cold skin, and other indications.

43. B: Auscultation is the method for taking an apical pulse, whereas A is the method for taking a peripheral pulse. D is wrong because both methods count for 30 seconds (multiplied by 2) for a regular heart rate or 60 seconds for an irregular rate. Gentle pressure (C) is used for taking a peripheral, not an apical, pulse.

44. D: This is the definition of negligence. If you were a doctor or other professional who must have a license in order to practice, you could also be sued for malpractice (B); nursing assistants cannot be sued for malpractice since they only need to maintain certification. Neglect (C) refers to harm subsequent to the accidental or deliberate ignoring of patient needs. Defamation (A) is the making of damaging statements about another individual.

45. C: Only Catholics and other Christians typically include pork in their diet. Muslims (A) and Jews (B) typically do not, and Hindus (D) are generally vegetarians or vegans. These cultural differences should be respected when ordering meals.

46. C: This is a violation of the first principle of good body mechanics, which is to retain a proper center of gravity by bending and lifting using the legs, not by bending over. The other answers comprise the other three principles of good body mechanics.

47. C: The nursing assistant should only discuss procedures that are within his/her own scope of practice, not any of the other choices. If family members have questions about the patient's overall care (D), they should be referred to the supervising nurse.

48. A: Of the choices, this is the only one where you do not need to have done proper hand washing, but once you plan to start a procedure such as feeding (B) you need to wash your hands. Anytime you could have been exposed to microorganisms, such as when using the restroom (C), eating, sneezing, or touching blood or body fluids—even if wearing gloves (D)—you should wash your hands.

49. C: At least 75 hours of classroom and basic skills training along with passing a written examination and skills demonstration are required in most states to be a CNA. Unspecified on-the-job training is not enough.

50. B: An NPO diet means that the patient should not be given any food or drink by mouth. It is one type of therapeutic or prescribed diet based on health issues, as are the other listed alternatives: a calorie-count diet for diabetics (A), a low-sodium diet for those with hypertension or renal problems (C), and a mechanical soft diet for people who cannot chew, such as those without teeth.

51. A: This is the correct sequence. All the other responses leave out essential components of infection control.

52. C: These symptoms are indications of possible deep vein thrombosis (DVT). The goal in this case is to prevent blood clots and to promote blood flow by applying pressure to the legs with a sequential compression device (A) or anti-embolism stockings (D). Anticoagulant therapy is a common treatment and surgery is performed if necessary (B). Massaging the leg (C), however, might dislodge a clot and lead to a heart attack or other serious complications.

53. B: If the patient is alert and capable of making decisions, you should not try to intervene (C) but refer him/her to the charge nurse. If the nurse cannot dissuade the patient, he/she is free to leave but the doctor should be notified. The patient may be asked to sign an Against Medical Advice form (A), but that is not your responsibility. Family members might be contacted, but ultimately the patient's decision to leave is his/her responsibility alone.

54. C: Dark, tarry stools are generally an indication of intestinal bleeding, not diarrhea (A), constipation (B), or dehydration (D).

55. B: This is the definition of empathy. All of the responses, however, are good tools for communicating with a patient. Active listening (A) is listening attentively while conversing, caring (C) is having genuine regard for the patient's safety and welfare, and respect (D) is showing consideration and regard for the patient's values.

56. C: This is the only correct combination.

57. B: The body should be washed, the perineal area covered, and a clean gown applied, but some other aspects of hygiene and grooming are unnecessary. Rigor mortis, the stiffening of muscles that occurs after death, makes limbs difficult to move, so placing the patient in a supine position (C) as soon as possible will make other postmortem tasks easier. All of the other responses are things that should be included in postmortem care.

58. B: Answer A is technically correct as long as the individual does not lose consciousness, but you should be aware of the possible need for rescue breathing and/or CPR. Gentle thrusts (C) may not dislodge the item, and you should not wait for emergency services (D).

59. D: A Patient's Bill of Rights is a listing of his/her rights while in the facility; it is specific to the facility but generally covers rights such as privacy, confidentiality, respectful care, etc. Patients generally get a list of responsibilities (C) when admitted but that is a different issue. There is a federal act governing privacy of health-care information (B) called HIPAA or Health Insurance Portability and Accountability Act.

60. B: A tort is damage committed for which restitution is generally awarded in a civil case, which excludes both C and D as they are considered criminal offenses. There are two types of torts: unintentional (B), in which the offender did not intend to cause harm; and intentional (A), in which the offender acts in a manner that he/she knows could result in harm.

61. A: You should always wash the perineal area of a female patient from front to back, rinse, and dry from front to back. The perineum extends from the vaginal opening to the anus. The other responses are incorrect.

62. A: Other than merely not getting along well with the patient, all of the other scenarios are justifiable reasons for refusing an assignment.

63. C: These are symptoms that the patient currently has low blood sugar (hypoglycemia) as opposed to those listed in (A) indicating hyperglycemia. The patient could become confused (B) from either abnormality, and excessive thirst (D) is a general sign of diabetes.

64. C: You should always strive to use terms that are the most respectful with regard to an impairment. All of the other choices could be considered demeaning.

65. B: When measuring input and output (I & O), input should include liquid food or other types of liquid intake, and output should include all fluids secreted. The primary output that is measurable is urine, but loss in other forms such as fluid in stool or vomit should also be estimated. Quantities should be logged in mL or cc, not ounces.

66. C: Valuable items such as dentures or hearing aids that patients will need on a daily basis can be kept in a box alongside the bed, but valuable jewelry should not be kept there. It should be sent home with a family member (A) or catalogued and stored in the facility safe (B), and you should only handle it in the presence of a witness (D).

67. B: The arm should be at the level of the heart throughout the measurement. Blood pressure is recorded as the systolic pressure (during contraction of the heart) over the diastolic pressure (when heart chambers are filling and at rest).

68. D: Continuity of care is a patient's right, and its components are both continuous and consistent high-quality care. The other choices do not ensure one of these components.

69. B: The four-point technique, which always maintains at least three points of contact with the floor, would be best since it ensures the most stability. The three-point technique (A) is useful for patients who cannot bear weight on one foot. Both swing methods (C and D) are not ideal because they require significant upper body strength.

70. C: A tub bath should be performed near the maximum temperature for bathing, which is 115°F. The acceptable range for a bed bath is 105°F to 115°F.

Practice Test 2

Practice Questions

1. The team member responsible for the policies, procedures, and actions of other team members while caring for a resident is the:
   a. Registered nurse (RN)
   b. Physical therapist
   c. Director of Nursing
   d. Licensed practical nurse (LPN)

2. Health care institutions may be designed to perform all of the following functions EXCEPT:
   a. Prevent disease and promote wellness
   b. Promote research
   c. Provide care to the ill or injured
   d. Profit and educate the business world

3. The team member responsible for writing and signing orders for medications and treatments is the:
   a. Physician or nurse practitioner
   b. LPN
   c. Administrator
   d. RN

4. Which facility best provides 24-hour nursing care to a client who is being discharged from an acute care facility but still requires around-the-clock care?
   a. Hospice
   b. Skilled nursing
   c. Assisted living
   d. Home care

5. All of the following are terms referring to the person being cared for EXCEPT:
   a. Client
   b. Resident
   c. Nursing assistant
   d. Patient

6. The team member responsible for providing supervision over all the other team members giving direct patient care is the:
   a. Nursing supervisor
   b. LPN
   c. Nurse practitioner
   d. RN

7. A complaint from a resident to the nursing assistant should be reported. To whom would the nursing assistant report complaints?
    a. The nursing assistant need not report the complaint to anyone if it is minor
    b. The complaints should be reported to the administrator first
    c. The complaints should be reported to the team leader
    d. The complaints should be reported to the physician

8. The definition of prognosis is best described as:
    a. A medical estimate of outcome for the disease process
    b. The date of expected death
    c. The reason for admission
    d. The type of behavior plan a resident is on

9. What is the best description of an administrator's primary function?
    a. Supervises nursing staff
    b. Handles only the money side of the facility
    c. Responsible for the entire operation of a facility
    d. Has no real responsibility but is required to be present by state regulations

10. The term for providing services for the terminally ill client is:
    a. Skilled care
    b. Home care
    c. Intermediate care
    d. Hospice care

11. Which selection is NOT the responsibility of a nursing assistant?
    a. Assisting a client with bathing
    b. Assisting with oral hygiene
    c. Supervising nursing staff
    d. Assisting residents with meals

12. How frequently should a CNA be responsible for mouth care of an unconscious client?
    a. Two times per shift
    b. Every two hours
    c. Every day
    d. Three times per shift

13. The appropriate way to store the dentures of a resident should include:
    a. It is not a task of the CNA.
    b. Consideration for the resident's preferences
    c. Placing dentures in a denture cup with cold water labeled with the client's name
    d. Sterilizing them in hot water

14. What is an action a nursing assistant may perform to make trimming the nails of an elderly resident easier?
    a. Nursing assistants will never perform nail care
    b. Soaking the nails in warm water first
    c. Painting the nails with clear polish before filing
    d. Buffing the nails for a sheen first

15. What is the most appropriate way for a nursing assistant to prevent the spread of infection?
    a. Using the autoclave for all equipment
    b. Washing hands between each resident's care
    c. Washing hands before and after each task
    d. Washing hands once a shift

16. All of the following should be reported to the charge nurse EXCEPT:
    a. Cooperative residents
    b. A resident sitting in wet clothing
    c. A resident complaining of constipation
    d. A new area of redness on the buttocks of a resident

17. A diabetic resident would be expected to have which type of diet?
    a. Low sodium
    b. High residue
    c. Sugar free
    d. Low fat

18. Seeing, feeling, and listening to a resident to gain data about the condition of the resident is an example of:
    a. Subjective data
    b. Objective observations
    c. Not a CNA responsibility
    d. Assumptions

19. The purpose of a thermometer is:
    a. To measure weight
    b. To take a blood pressure
    c. To determine body heat
    d. Record the pulse

20. A resident complains of pain and swelling in her ankle. What is the proper medical term for swelling?
    a. Bruise
    b. Analgesia
    c. Puffy
    d. Edema

21. What is the general medical term that would include proteins and carbohydrates?
    a. Food
    b. Nutrients
    c. Substance
    d. Enzymes

22. What piece of equipment being used on a resident would keep the nursing assistant from also using an electric razor during hygiene?
    a. Oxygen
    b. Heating pad
    c. Ice mattress
    d. Knee brace

23. Which response by the nursing assistant would be most appropriate when the hospice resident talks about dying?
    a. "I can't discuss this with you, but I will get a nurse."
    b. "You are not going to die today."
    c. "You have a wonderful doctor. I'm sure you will be feeling better soon."
    d. "How does this make you feel?"

24. Which would be the most appropriate action for the nursing assistant when a resident has large amounts of oral mucus?
    a. Suction aggressively to clear the throat
    b. Report excessive secretions to the physician
    c. Report the condition to the charge nurse
    d. Place a towel under the resident's chin

25. Which selection would not be considered a comfort measure for an elderly dying resident?
    a. Offering a back rub without turning the resident
    b. Repositioning the resident once a shift
    c. Turning and repositioning every two hours
    d. Allowing family members to leave the room when care is taking place

26. A resident who promises to stop smoking if only God will take his cancer away is displaying the stage of death and dying best termed as:
    a. Acceptance
    b. Denial
    c. Confusion
    d. Bargaining

27. The term describing the care given to a resident after death is referred to as:
    a. Comfort care
    b. Premortem care
    c. Postmortem care
    d. Quality care

28. The term for extremity and body stiffness after death is:
    a. Corpse
    b. Rigor mortis
    c. Arthritis
    d. Incontinence

29. The care given to a resident by a nurse or nursing assistant in the client's home is termed:
   a. Hospice
   b. Home health care
   c. Outpatient care
   d. Outpatient clinic care

30. To care for a client in their own home, the state requires which of the following for a nursing assistant?
   a. A nursing license
   b. A nursing assistant license
   c. A state certification
   d. Completion of an approved home health aide program

31. Which of the following selections best describes what qualifies a client for home health care services?
   a. Insurance
   b. A medical condition requiring medications or assessments
   c. Medicare only will determine home health care status.
   d. Being divorced or to living alone

32. Home health care may not be initiated without first:
   a. Obtaining consent from the next of kin
   b. Obtaining a physician order
   c. Obtaining a social service consult
   d. Obtaining payment status

33. Assisting with daily living tasks and light housekeeping may be required in the home health setting and will be provided by which professional?
   a. Nursing assistant
   b. Nurse
   c. Housekeeper
   d. Family members

34. Which statement best documents when a client is forgetful and confused at times?
   a. The client had a good day
   b. The client is forgetful and confused at times
   c. The client can be forgetful
   d. The client had a bad day

35. Which vital sign measurement would need immediate reporting to the charge nurse?
   a. Blood pressure of 120/60
   b. A heart rate of 78
   c. A temperature of 100.1° F
   d. A temperature of 104.1° F

36. Understanding cultural diversity includes all of the following selections except:
    a Believing all patients will have the same experiences
    b. Understanding that each resident may have a different set of religious beliefs
    c. Knowing that residents may have a variety of lifestyles
    d. Acknowledging that each resident may have different customs for holidays, meals, and social behaviors

37. What is the general term that refers to NOT discussing a resident with family, friends, or in public places?
    a. Rudeness
    b. Polite behavior
    c. Confidentiality
    d. Secretive professional behavior

38. Which of the following is NOT a responsibility of a nursing assistant when providing home health care to a client?
    a. Assisting with the bath
    b. Helping to brush the client's teeth
    c. Administering medications
    d. Helping a client to dress

39. Which artery is being measured when a blood pressure is taken in the upper arm?
    a. Brachial
    b. Radial
    c. Ulnar
    d. Carotid

40. Which device(s) will be used to monitor blood pressures?
    a. Cuff and thermometer
    b. Cuff and stethoscope
    c. Sphygmomanometer and thermometer
    d. None of the above

41. Which blood pressure reading should be reassessed and reported immediately to the charge nurse?
    a. 140/90
    b. 180/90
    c. 120/70
    d. 120/80

42. What is a normal heart rate at rest for an adult?
    a. 70
    b. 110
    c. 40
    d. 160

43. What devastating side effect may result from hypertension?
    a. Fainting
    b. Diabetes
    c. Cancer
    d. Stroke

44. Taking an oral temperature is appropriate for most clients EXCEPT:
    a. A teen with abdominal pain
    b. An elderly man on oxygen with emphysema
    c. A female who has not had a drink for one hour
    d. A 10-year-old who can hold her lips closed

45. What is the best artery to feel for a pulse when monitoring the pulse rate?
    a. Brachial
    b. Carotid
    c. Radial
    d. Pedal

46. Symptom(s) that should be reported to the nurse after doing oral hygiene with a resident include:
    a. White teeth
    b. Pink gums
    c. Pink moist tongue
    d. Dry cracked lips or tongue, bleeding gums

47. The nursing assistant assists the resident who is being admitted to the facility. Which action should the nursing assistant complete immediately following this?
    a. Call the physician
    b. Report the information to the charge nurse
    c. Call the pharmacy for medications
    d. The nursing assistant does not help with an admission

48. The resident states she has a diamond ring and ruby necklace on her person. What would the nursing assistant document when recording the belongings of this resident?
    a. Diamond ring, ruby necklace
    b. Ring, necklace
    c. Clear stone ring and red stone necklace
    d. None of the above

49. A resident who is nervous and uncooperative maybe feeling which emotions?
    a. Anxiety
    b. Fatigue
    c. Joy
    d. Coma

50. What is the most appropriate attire for a new admission to the nursing facility to wear during an assessment?
    a. A jogging suit
    b. Silk pajamas
    c. A hospital gown
    d. Street clothes of any kind

51. A resident is new to the facility and starts complaining of hunger and thirst. What is the appropriate action for the nursing assistant?
    a. To offer clear liquids and advance the diet as the resident tolerates it
    b. To place the client on puree foods initially
    c. To order a regular diet for the client
    d. To report the complaint to the charge nurse so diet orders may be obtained from the physician

52. The most appropriate way to address a new client is by:
    a. Calling him or her sweetie
    b. Calling him or her honey
    c. Using Mr. or Ms. and the last name
    d. Using the client's first name only without permission

53. What is the best time to begin discharge teaching and planning for a new resident?
    a. The day before discharge
    b. The week before discharge
    c. The day of admission
    d. When the client is receptive

54. Who writes the discharge order for a client?
    a. The LPN on duty
    b. The physician
    c. The social worker
    d. The case manager

55. The purpose of ROM exercises is:
    a. To prevent decubitus ulcers and contractures
    b. To promote weight loss
    c. To encourage the client to get well
    d. To prevent bruising and skin tears

56. The most important aspect of a bowel and bladder training program should be:
    a. Diet
    b. Offering the bedpan or bathroom every two hours
    c. High fluid intake
    d. Laxatives every few hours

57. The appropriate time frame to wash your hands between each task is:
    a. 1–2 minutes
    b. 3–4 minutes
    c. 30 seconds
    d. 5 minutes

58. The appropriate way to turn off the faucets after hand washing is:
    a. With gloves
    b. With soapy hands
    c. With paper towel
    d. With an elbow or knee

59. The areas to wash along with the hands should include:
    a. Washing up to the elbows
    b. Stopping at the wrists
    c. Six inches above the wrists
    d. Two inches above the wrists

60. The appropriate order of putting on isolations protection should be:
    a. Gown, mask, gloves
    b. Mask, gloves, gown
    c. Gown, gloves, mask
    d. Mask, gown, gloves

61. Which statement best describes a nursing assistant's understanding of proper glove application?
    a. Gloves are optional
    b. Gloves are to cover the cuffs of the gown
    c. Gloves do not cover the cuffs of the gown
    d. Gloves go on first

62. Isolation is initiated in order to:
    a. Keep the patient secluded
    b. Provide protection for visitors
    c. Provide protection to the resident and to the staff
    d. Provide protection to the physician making rounds

63. The appropriate treatment of linen in an isolation room would include:
    a. No special treatment is required
    b. Washing with hot soap and water
    c. Bagging the linen inside the room, then bagging or double bagging it outside the room with the help of a coworker
    d. Double bagging inside the room without an assistant

64. What is the proper placement of the mask as protective equipment?
    a. It should cover the mouth
    b. It should cover the mouth and nose
    c. It should cover the nose
    d. None of the above

65. Which piece of linen should be placed on the top of the pile when making a bed in a client's room?
    a. The draw sheet
    b. The top sheet
    c. The pillow cases
    d. The bottom sheet

66. Which action is most appropriate when making the bed of a resident and will aide in preventing skin breakdown?
    a. Making sure the bottom sheet is slightly moist
    b. Making sure the top sheet is tightly secured
    c. Making sure the bottom sheet is wrinkle free
    d. None of the above

67. Which action is most appropriate when placing the sheets on the bed to prevent the spread of organisms into the air?
    a. Use sterile sheets
    b. Lay the sheet on the bed and unfold carefully without shaking
    c. Shaking the sheets to spread them evenly
    d. No special way is required

68. What is one way to keep sheets secured to the foot of the bed for a client?
    a. Folding and tucking with a mitered corner at the foot of the bed
    b. Tape them to the mattress
    c. Tie them to the bed frame
    d. There is no special way to secure sheets or to keep them secure for a client

69. What is the most appropriate head position when doing oral care on an unconscious client?
    a. Placing the head midline with the eyes looking to the ceiling
    b. The head to the right only
    c. The head to the left only
    d. Position the head to the right or left side

70. Which is the most appropriate way to give oral hygiene to an unconscious resident?
    a. A toothbrush and water
    b. With oral glycerin swabs
    c. With a syringe and mouthwash
    d. It is not necessary to do oral care for an unconscious client

Answers and Explanations

1. C: The Director of Nursing is responsible for the policies and procedures that govern how a resident is cared for in a facility. She or he is also responsible for making certain that all team members are educated and trained to properly care for residents and that there are team members in place to provide adequate supervision. The Director of Nursing is at the top of the chain of command and reports to the Administrator.

2. D: The purpose of any healthcare institution will center on promoting wellness, preventing disease, providing research, and providing care to the ill or injured. The main purpose of a health institution should always be related to the client's well-being and health. There is a business side to running every healthcare institution, but their purpose is not to educate for profit. Healthcare institutions are instead in the business of caring for clients or providing research into health and disease.

3. A: The physician or nurse practitioner is the team member who writes orders for medications and treatments. An RN may take a verbal/telephone order for a medication, but the order must be signed by the physician or NPN within hours of giving the order.

4. B: Skilled nursing facilities provide 24-hour nursing care with a nurse on duty 24 hours and the majority of care being provided by nursing assistants. Hospice is for end of life and palliative care. Home care is not 24-hour care and depends on the family to provide some of the care. Assisted living requires the resident to be somewhat self sufficient.

5. C: The person being cared for may be referred to as the client, the patient, or the resident, depending on the facility and their preferred terminology. The nursing assistant is the person giving the care, and therefore the exception.

6. A: The nursing supervisor is responsible for overseeing all the care given by the other team members. It may be the same RN on staff for a given shift, but most often there is a nursing supervisor who oversees the entire team, including the shift RN, LPN, and nursing assistant.

7. C: Complaints should always be brought to the attention of the team leader. The team leader has the skills necessary to be professional and to address the complaint in the appropriate manner. A nursing assistant is not responsible for notifying the physician or the administrator with patient complaints. All complaints should be mentioned to the team leader.

8. A: The prognosis is the best guess for an expected outcome based on medical knowledge of the disease process. The other choices are incorrect. No one can actually estimate date of death with any certainty (b). Also, reason for admission (c) would be tied to the patient's diagnosis and its prognosis, but is not the definition for either term, nor is the treatment plan (d).

9. C: The administrator is responsible for the entire operation of a facility. He or she must meet with all the department heads on a regular basis to ensure that the facility is running smoothly. The other choices are facets of the administrator's responsibility but not the entirety and are, therefore, incorrect.

10. D: The term for care provided for the terminally ill client is hospice. Intermediate care (c) is provided with unlicensed caregivers and licensed supervisors. Home care (b) is care partially given by licensed or unlicensed nursing assistants or nurses and partially given by family members. To be considered skilled nursing care a., services must be provided by an RN or by an LPN under the supervision of an RN. Hospice care may be provided in a client's own home for pain and comfort, but most of the care is provided by family. Hospice in this situation, however, refers to the type of care given at a special facility or in a special way to give care and comfort to the client who is not expected to live much longer.

11. C: The nursing assistant will not be responsible for supervising nursing staff. A nursing assistant may help to precept or orient new nursing assistants but the RN is responsible for supervising nursing staff while the director of nursing is absent or in the absence of a nursing supervisor. The daily tasks for care are the responsibilities of the nursing assistant.

12. B: The client who is unconscious should have oral care every two hours to keep mucous membranes moist and to prevent skin breakdown.

13. C: The proper way to care for dentures is to place them in a cup filled with cold water, labeled with the client's name. It is also appropriate to clean the dentures and return them to the client's mouth. Since denture care may, indeed, be one of the CNA's tasks, answer a. is incorrect. Although patient preferences are important (b), they may not always be compatible with standard processes for care. Sterilizing dentures (d) is not a regular responsibility for the CNA.

14. B: Nursing assistants may be asked to file or trim fingernails of the residents, and soaking in warm water prior to trimming makes it easier and safer. The nails of the elderly become hard and brittle and soaking softens the nail for trimming.

15. C: is the most appropriate way to prevent the spread of infection. Washing hands before a task and after a task protects the CNA, as well as the resident.

16. A: Cooperative residents are a pleasure, not a symptom, and therefore need not be reported to the charge nurse. The other choices may need a nursing intervention, so they should always be reported.

17. C: Diabetes is related to sugar and insulin production. A sugar free diet is therefore appropriate. The other diets are not directly related to diabetic care.

18. B: Objective observations involve seeing, feeling, or listening, and what is discovered may be reported to the nurse in charge, if needed. CNAs do learn to assess for symptoms that may need to be reported to the RN or LPN in charge.

19. C: The thermometer determines what the body temperature of the resident is. Conversely, a scale is used to measure weight a., a blood pressure cuff is used for blood pressure readings (b), and pulse checks (d) are often done manually.

20. D: The proper medical term for swelling is edema.

21. B: Nutrients include carbohydrates and proteins and may be in foods, formula, parental nutrition, and tube feeding mixtures.

22. A: A resident who uses oxygen should not also use an electric razor because of the risk of sparks from the razor. The heating pad (b) may be discontinued while shaving, as can the ice mattress (c). A knee brace (d) poses no risk.

23. D: Allowing residents to discuss their feelings will be more beneficial than having the nursing assistant ignore or refuse. A charge nurse may be asked to also help with the discussion, but the most important thing is to listen.

24. C: Reporting to the charge nurse is most appropriate, so the nurse can come to suction and assess. Placing a towel may be appropriate as well, but it doesn't take the place of reporting to the nurse in charge.

25. C: It is important for comfort to turn the resident every two hours and simultaneously reposition. Once a shift is not enough, and a back rub without turning and repositioning is not effective. Family members may or may not feel comfortable assisting with care.

26. D: Bargaining is the stage of death and dying where the resident begins promising a particular behavior in exchange for wellness.

27. C: Postmortem care is the care given after the resident or client dies. "Post" means after, and "mortem" means death.

28. B: Rigor mortis is the stiffening of the body after death. It is appropriate to close the eyelids, use care with positioning the hands of the victim, and attempt to close the mouth so the face and hands take on a more natural appearance for the funeral director and his tasks.

29. B: Home health care is the proper term for any health care provided in the home of the client. It may or may not be hospice care as well, depending on the diagnosis and prognosis for the client.

30. D: The home health nursing assistant must complete an approved home health aid program that teaches the skills needed to provide care for a resident in the home setting.

31. B: The patient must have a medical condition that requires medication or assessments by a skilled professional in order to qualify for home health care.

32. B: Obtaining a physician order is a requirement for beginning home health care. The other selections may or may not take place, but they are not required for home health care to be established.

33. A: The tasks described are within the scope of work of a nursing assistant.

34. B: "The client is forgetful and confused at times" best describes how it should be documented. It is specific and pertinent. The other options are either insufficiently specific, as with (c), or lacking any reference to the client's problem, as with a. and (d).

35. D: A temperature of 104.1° F is extremely high and would need to be reported, so the charge nurse could provide the proper intervention.

36. A: When you believe that all residents have the same experiences, you do not understand the differences in each culture or, indeed, in each individual. The other selections all show a basic understanding of some of the differences that may occur in a variety of cultures.

37. C: Confidentiality is the term for refusing to discuss clients outside of a professional need-to-know basis.

38. C: It is not within the scope of practice for a nursing assistant to administer medications unless they have been certified to do so. It would be the responsibility of a nurse, family member, or qualified medication aide to administer medications.

39. A: The brachial artery is the artery used when taking a blood pressure in the upper arm. The radial artery is for taking a pulse in the wrist. The ulnar artery is deeper and may sometimes be palpated in the wrist as well. The carotid artery may be palpated in the neck but is not used for a blood pressure.

40. B: The stethoscope is used for listening along with the blood pressure cuff to measure and monitor the blood pressure. The sphygmomanometer is also used but not with a thermometer.

41. B: A blood pressure of 180/90 is too high and should be reported to the charge nurse for possible intervention. A blood pressure of 140/90 is high normal and should be reported at some point in time, but it does not necessarily need an immediate intervention. The other two readings fall within the normal range.

42. A: A normal adult heart rate is 70–100 beats per minute.

43. D: Stroke is one of the most serious side effects of hypertension or high blood pressure. Fainting may occur in relation to a spike in blood pressure but is not normally "devastating." Diabetes is not a side effect of high blood pressure, nor is cancer.

44. B: A client on oxygen cannot hold the thermometer in a closed lip position, and the oxygen may alter the client's temperature, depending on how high the flow is and whether it is being heated.

45. C: The radial artery is in the wrist and is the location at which a pulse is most often measured.

46. D: A dry cracked tongue or lips and bleeding gums indicate dehydration and poor oral hygiene. The nurse should be informed, so an intervention may be initiated. The other selections are normal for a healthy mouth.

47. B: The nursing assistant does not call the doctor or pharmacy, but she or he does help do admissions and would report relevant admissions information to the charge nurse.

48. C: The nursing assistant has no way of knowing if the ring and necklace are real diamond and ruby or imitation, so the color of the stones should be described, rather than assuming the jewelry is real.

49. A: The nursing assistant should understand that the resident may be feeling anxiety. The symptoms should also be reported to the charge nurse, so an assessment may be made to determine if there is a medical reason for the behavior.

50. C: A hospital gown allows for a complete assessment of the condition of the resident's skin.

51. D: The nursing assistant must report the symptoms of hunger and thirst to a nurse, so the appropriate diet can be ordered and to determine whether the resident may have food or drink in the meantime.

52. C: The appropriate way to address a client is to show respect by using Mr. or Ms. and the client's last name.

53. C: The day of admission is the time to start thinking about discharge and what information needs to be addressed with the client.

54. B: The physician will write the order approving discharge for a client.

55. A: The purpose of moving the client and doing range of motion exercises is to prevent decubitus ulcers and contractures.

56. B: Although all the selections may have their place in a bowel and bladder training program, the most important aspect is to offer the bedpan or bathroom every two hours.

57. A: Hand washing should take a minute or longer each time.

58. C: The best way to turn off the water is to use the paper towel you have dried with and then discard it.

59. D: Wash your hands and up to two inches above the wrists to remove all bacteria between each task.

60. A: When putting on protective equipment, put on your gown first, followed by the mask, and finish with the gloves up over the cuffs of the gown.

61. B: The gloves go over the cuffs of the gown to protect the wrists from bacteria and contaminants.

62. C: Isolation protects the client, as well as the staff.

63. C: The linen should be bagged inside the room and then double bagged outside the room with the help of another person.

64. B: The mask covers the mouth and nose.

65. D: The bottom sheet will be used first so it should be on the top of the pile. Layering the linen in the order of use decreases the chances of dropping it on the floor and contaminating it in other ways.

66. C: The bottom sheet should be wrinkle free to help avoid skin irritation or breakdown for the resident.

67. B: Lay the sheet on the bed and unfold it carefully to keep from shaking and spreading airborne germs.

68. A: Tucking the corners in a mitered fashion keeps the covers secure and helps the client to keep covered without dropping loose linen to the floor.

69. D: When the client is unconscious, it is most appropriate to position the head to the side—to the right or to the left—to assist with oral secretions and to avoid choking hazards for the client.

70. B: The best way to give oral hygiene to an unconscious patient is with oral glycerin swabs made especially for mouth care. It helps to moisten the mouth and aids in the prevention of sores.